FLU PANDEMIC OF 2018-2019

How Can We Learn From The Spanish Flu Epidemic of 1918 And Prepare for What's Coming

D.W. Graeme

Copyright 2018 by D.W. Graeme

All rights Reserved. No part of this book may be reproduced in any form without permission in writing from the author. Reviewers may quote brief passages in reviews.

The following Book is reproduced below with the goal of providing information that is as accurate and reliable as possible. Regardless, purchasing this Book can be seen as consent to the fact that both the publisher and the author of this book are in no way experts on the topics discussed within and that any recommendations or suggestions that are made herein are for entertainment purposes only.

Professionals should be consulted as needed prior to undertaking any of the action endorsed herein.

This declaration is deemed fair and valid by both the American Bar Association and the Committee of Publishers Association and is legally binding throughout the United States.

Furthermore, the transmission, duplication or reproduction of any of the following work including specific information will be considered an illegal act irrespective of if it is done electronically or in print.

This extends to creating a secondary or tertiary copy of the work or a recorded copy and is only allowed with express written consent from the Publisher. All additional right reserved.

The information in the following pages is broadly considered to be a truthful and accurate account of facts and as such any inattention, use or misuse of the *information in question by the reader will render any resulting actions solely under their purview. There are no scenarios in which the publisher or the original author of this work can be in any fashion deemed liable for any hardship or damages that may befall them after undertaking information described herein.*

Additionally, the information in the following pages is intended only for informational purposes and should thus be thought of as universal. As befitting its nature, it is presented without assurance regarding its prolonged validity or interim quality. Trademarks that are mentioned are done without written consent and can in no way be considered an endorsement from the trademark holder.

FLU PANDEMIC OF 2018-2019: How Can We Learn From the Spanish Flu Epidemic of 1918 and Prepare for What's Coming

Table of Contents

Introduction 6

Chapter One:
What Do We Know From The Spanish Flu Epidemic of 1918? 8

Chapter Two:
So, Who Were the Survivors of the Flu Epidemic of 1918, and Why? 13

Chapter Three:
But, How Did The Flu Epidemic of 1918 Spread? 22

Chapter Four:
1976 Swine Flu Pandemic Scare 32

Chapter Five:
Why World Health Authorities Are Now Worried About The Next Flu Pandemic 41

Chapter Six:
Where, When, And How Will The Next Major Flu Epidemic Hit Us? 48

Chapter Seven:
The Department Of Defense During A Flu Pandemic 62

Chapter Eight:
So, How Do We Move Forward? 65

Final Words 76

Introduction

This book will tell you what happened in 1918 when the Flu Pandemic went around the world killing millions, but in the United States alone it killed 675,000.

Scientists tell us that we are due for another Pandemic and they predict it will be in later in 2018 & 2019. They fear it will come from China and the open-air poultry markets and make its way quickly across the planet killing as it comes across the globe.

It takes six months to develop a flu vaccine and not knowing which strain the Pandemic will bring with it; it will be almost impossible to be prepared with a vaccine for the citizens of all countries.

We need to look at how it will affect our countries financially and how to protect our families and ourselves 'when' not 'if' this Pandemic comes our way.

It will give you examples of families and some of their trials and losses they encountered in 1918 and 2017.

This book should help you to understand the flu virus itself and why developing the vaccine is so hard and what is standing in its way. It will explain that the science is there; but the paperwork, the trials, the red tape, the marketing and possibly Big

Pharma (being against) to make a universal vaccine that is given once every ten years is standing in the way.

I hope that when you finish this book, you will have a better idea of how to protect your family and yourself when the Pandemic sweeps across the Globe.

Chapter One: What Do We Know From The Spanish Flu Epidemic of 1918?

1918 had to be considered a terrible and sad year for our forefathers. Hopeful soldiers were so glad to be returning from WWI. They were coming home to their families and loved ones in hopes to see their fiances, and children. Instead, they were coming back and being greeted by one of the worst pandemics ever to hit the modern day World.

They did not know at the time they were part of the problem because they did not realize the flu had followed them home. During this time there was so little known about how the flu was being transferred between humans or some other source because it had not yet been identified.

The one thing that everyone did know was that people were dying at such a rapid rate it was unbelievable. You might be feeling fine one day, and within 36 hours you were dead, and whatever it was, it was spreading like wildfire.

The Spanish Flu Pandemic of 1918 was not

handled well by our government and the public health department at the time. The United States did not want it to be known so that our soldiers would not find out while they were fighting in WWI so their morale would not break down. Since Spain was not at war, they started spreading the word for us. When word got out, the flu had been said to come from Spain; it became dubbed as the Spanish Flu when it never was the Spanish Flu.

It was in 1917 the United States Government passed a law. It started with the President at the time, Woodrow Wilson. This law stated if anyone were to "print, publish, utter, or write anything that was profane, disloyal, scurrilous, profane, or had any abusive language in it about the United States government they could receive punishment by up to 20 years in prison. For those who spoke their mind that was probably an excellent deterrent to not say a thing.

What was stranger still, as the flu approached the next city or town, the officials of the city were told to tell the people of the town or city not to worry, that the health officials had it all under control and no one there would be affected. When the flu hit the city, the town officials would tell the townspeople that it was just the ordinary flu and no way it was the Spanish flu. As it exploded in their faces, the town officials kept telling the townspeople the worst was all but over.

For some reason, the town officials thought they were more educated than any of the townspeople. They felt that they should lie to keep the people from being scared since, in their opinion, worry killed more folks than the epidemic would ever kill. (Robertson, 1918) I am not sure what rock he crawled out from under, but he certainly had no grasp on how to handle the public and be truthful.

In the city of Brotherly Love, Philadelphia, it was none other but the Public Health Commissioner that decided to close all houses of worship, public gathering places, closed all the schools, and theaters. The Commissioner would follow this announcement at the end, "but you don't need to worry or be alarmed." What a crock he was spreading when everyone was aware of all those who lived around them dying terrible, horrendous deaths.

In the city of Chicago, in the County Hospital, the flu mortality rate was at 39.8%.

Back in Philadelphia, dead bodies were not being picked up from homes for days. Eventually, they would send trucks with open beds and some horse-drawn carts down the streets. Families were told to bring their dead out to the street. There were so many dead that they just stacked them without coffins and all they could do was bury them in mass graves in cemeteries by using steam shovels. How sad for the family members. My heart cannot imagine what those living must have felt.

My grandmother always had a saying that seems so right in most all cases of death and dying. It went something like this, "Living troubles are worse than dead troubles." If you think about what grandma said for a minute, this is so true. Those who have stepped out into Eternity, their troubles are over. No more sickness and sorrow, but the living still must face what might happen tomorrow, and for those living during the Pandemic, they did not know what would meet them the next minute.

The people affected heard what the public officials said but did not know what was really happening, and they had no one to trust for the real facts. They did not know what was happening in their own town except what they saw out their windows, let alone around the United States or the World.

People starved to death during this time. They were too sick to prepare themselves food. There was no fast food or canned goods to eat at that time, so everything had to be prepared over a wood fire. The sick were so sick that they just had no energy or were so riddled with a high fever they could not even get out of bed, and they starved to death because their neighbors were afraid to enter their homes to help them.

Chapter Two:
So, Who Were the Survivors of the Flu Epidemic of 1918, and Why?

Here are some people at the time, who survived and a brief account of what happened.

Edvard Munch, a famous Norwegian artist, known for his most famous work 'The Scream." This picture was painted as he tried to come to grips with his sister's mental illness.

After he was ill with the flu in 1918, he painted a self-portrait of his suffering. His face is pale, he looks very frail, and he is sitting all wrapped up in his dressing gown. He sits with his mouth wide open to show how tortured he is by his sickly state.

Woodrow Wilson, (President of the US at the time) was another matter entirely. President's physicians being used to hiding the illnesses of the presidents, always acted like it was nothing. It is what they do even now. What was happening after Woodrow's stroke that he suffered, his second wife acted in his place as President because they were hiding her husband from other political officials and the public.

As if having a stroke was not enough, he came down with 'the flu' while he was at a Peace Conference in Versailles during March or April of 1919. People noticed he was confused at times and he finally told his doctor that he felt terrible and was having trouble breathing. His temperature when they checked was 103 degrees. The physician told the press that the president had a cold. He had been around many at the conference who had all been in contact with him while he was most contagious, where he could contaminate all who were near him.

<u>Franklin Delano Roosevelt</u> seemed only to be affected by Polio and was a future president. When the end of World War I was coming to an end, since Franklin Delano Roosevelt was then the Assistant Secretary to the Navy, he was persuaded to travel to France. His fifth cousin, "Teddy," former President of the US said he should do this and meet with French officials and the "front line" troops.

On his way back home on the USS Leviathan, there were several on board the ship that had influenza from the pandemic. Several of them dying while on the vessel. FDR didn't just get the flu, but he also came down with double pneumonia. He was so overcome with the illness that he could not even walk off the ship, but they had to carry him off on a stretcher.

General John J. Pershing who was dubbed General "Black Jack" Pershing, led our American Forces in late September 1918 was calling for reinforcements because his men were dropping like flies from the Pandemic, and he needed more men for part of a significant military endeavor. The next call he made was for 142,000 men. They told him, we can't do it. We have had to stop all draft calls and stayed all training because of the Spanish Flu.

The conditions were so severe that even General Pershing came down with the virus. He was so sick and even delirious that he made some wrong decisions during the first days of November 1918. He had written a long letter to the War Council about negotiating peace, and it seemed like he was about to abandon his trying to move toward Armistice. Whatever went down, on November 11, 2018, WW1 was over.

Kaiser Wilhelm II has been the center of some conspiracy theories including that the Kaiser himself was the one who was responsible for the influenza pandemic. Some even say that he ordered the German U-Boats to poison Boston Harbor with the virus. He did however help instigate all of WWI, which did spread the flu itself.

The Kaiser also had a severe case of the flu in 1908, and they think he had it again in 1918. We well know now that it could not have been the same strain of flu both years. By November 28, 1918, he had no support of his army, so he left his post of Emperor.

Georgia O'Keeffe who was a famous American artist that was most known for her paintings of New York skyscrapers. She held her first New York solo exhibition and Alfred Stieglitz, a gallery owner, hosted her.

O'Keeffe was in Texas teaching when the flu caught up with her in the spring of 1919. At that time, their relationship was more than friends and Stieglitz was still married to his wife of twenty-five years. Even though he was twenty years older than O'Keeffe, Alfred convinced her to come back to New York to get well in his Manhattan home.

Mary Pickford was America's movie icon sweetheart. She came down with the flu in January of 1919. Her recovery progress was followed closely in all the newspapers.

Katherine Anne Porter was a Pulitzer Prize-winning author. While she was working as a journalist in 1918, she became a victim of the flu.

Katherine was already very ill with bronchitis, or so they thought, but she was misdiagnosed. However, this brought her to write a short novel, "Pale Horse, Pale Rider." It is a journalist who is in love with a soldier. The journalist gets very ill with the flu and is delirious. The soldier takes care of her, and when she gets well, she finds out that the love of her life died of the flu.

She goes on to write that the journalist is depressed once she recovers from the flu. As for Porter, having the flu, it seems to have caused her hair to turn grey and stayed that way.

<u>Walt Disney</u> came down with the flu in September 1918. At age 17, he was eager to sign up and serve his country. His buddy was turned down, and since they both wanted to stay together, they decided to join the Red Cross Ambulance Corps. Their first assignment was to go to training on the south side of Chicago, and that is where Walt came down full force with the flu. He went back home to be taken care of by his mother and rejoined the Corps in December.

When Walt arrived in France with the Red Cross, he could not believe the suffering, the illnesses, and evidence everywhere of war. This experience alone matured him more than anyone could ever know, and he was looking forward to going home.

There was another soldier who I knew very well. I did not come to meet him until many years later. It was my fraternal grandfather. A man I admired more than words can express. He had told me many times of the flu pandemic of 1918, and he never understood how he and his sisters survived it.

How I wish he were here now, so I could explain it to him.

I would be able to tell Grandpa that there was a milder strain of the same flu that came around in the spring of 1918 that some people caught and recovered. Most thought it was a slight, aggravating cold or allergies that spring. An aggravating sniffle and cough, so to speak, that usually lasted about three days.

Those who had caught this mild strain were some of the luckiest people in the world.

This light strain had given them 'active immunity' to the flu so that when they were exposed to the 'bad strain' of it that fall, they did not succumb to the illness nor show any signs or symptoms.

The pandemic must have stayed on grandpa's mind a lot because he seemed to talk about it often or maybe the seriousness of it has just stuck in my mind so much after all he had been through in his life. As a young man, he had just returned from the war. He had been on a mine destroyer in the North Seas.

After returning home to the family farm, he said he would wake up in the morning and until it turned dark he was burying people. He buried so many friends, neighbors, and strangers that all of their faces were just a blur. They did not even have time to build coffins for them nor have a decent funeral as the family was too sick to plan or attend the funeral. Most of the bodies they just wrapped in sheets or blankets, quilts, or whatever the family could find to wrap them in before they lay them in the ground. It was not a one or two-day event either. It went on for weeks on end. Remember this flu pandemic lasted through the spring of 1919. He said he had never dug that many graves for so many for something so sad.

My family was no more special than any other family of that period, but my grandfather believed in always helping your neighbor, and that was not just those who lived over on the next farm.

People of that time had to face a lot of sadness. They seemed more stoic emotionally than what we are now. I am not talking about just my forefathers, but all forefathers of our country.

For the others who survived, it depended on their age in life and their immune status. If they were very young and had not developed any antibodies yet, they were immediately victims. The very old more than likely had the antibodies but usually not a strong immune system. The young adults more than likely had not been exposed to the flu strain yet and had not developed the antibodies to ward off the flu, but they had a robust immune system that they would soon find out would not be in their favor.

Anyone who was immuno-compromised for any reason was more than likely to succumb to the flu and more than likely to be a statistic in the death toll.

I can tell you that for many, homeopathy was a considerable success in treating Swine Flu in 1918. Mortality rates for those who were treated by traditional drugs were 30-40%, but those who had a doctor who treated them with homeopathic remedies had a mortality rate of only 1.05%. It was staggering and mind-boggling.

There were cases treated at the Homeopathic Hospital in Washington D.C., and the recoveries were 100%.

The homeopathic remedies that were used during the trying time of the Great Flu Pandemic of 1918 were Bryonia and Gelsemium. Dr. Frank

Wieland from Chicago said they had 8,000 workers and had only one death and Gelsemium was the only drug they used. They did not use any vaccines, nor did they use aspirin.

For sure Homeopathy was successful 98% of the time in 1918.

What does this say for future pandemics? I know what it tells me. You will have to make up your mind for yourself.

Many stories validate treating with homeopathic treatments and all of them being successful in the research literature. It is the same success story every time. The working mechanism as to how it affects the virus I have not been able to find. I have an idea - It has something to do with stopping the replication of the virus itself.

The bottom line for the affected patients that were survivors like my grandfather were those who contracted the Pandemic strain of the flu of 1918 in that you had developed a light case in the spring of that year and had developed antibodies for the virulent strain that presented itself that Fall.

Or, you found yourself lucky enough to be taken care of by a homeopathic physician and were given the homeopathic drugs.

Chapter Three: But, How Did The Flu Epidemic of 1918 Spread?

There is some argument as to where the flu started. I cannot imagine who would want to admit that it began in their country, but there are many ideas as to where it did start.

The Flu Pandemic of 1918 killed 50 to 100 million worldwide.

Due to inadequate bookkeeping in some of the remote countries knows for sure the real number. We will never know an accurate figure for some of the countries. It had managed to kill more people in one year than the bubonic plague has killed in a century. The Pandemic of 1918 lasted for 15 months, but if you lived it, it seemed to be years as it dragged on.

The pandemic killed 670,000 Americans in the United States alone.

Today, Americans become worried over Ebola, Zika, and other weird new exotic pathogens but do not worry about the flu. It is a big mistake that they do not pay more attention to the flu because one day they will wish they had paid more attention to all the facts.

Right now, we are in as much danger if not more than we were of another pandemic as they were in 1918. Public Health Officials will tell you that is our biggest threat we face health wise.

Let's look back at how the situation lay in 1918. It could explain a scenario in many small towns in America, but this one fits the bill the best as to where it started.

Let's start in Haskell County, Kansas in 1918, and most folks were still living in their sod houses.

Haskell farmers raise pigs (clue #1). (Clue #2) This same county also sits on a migratory flyway for not one, not two, but 17 different bird species, making it a major migratory flyway. The birds include mallards and sand hill cranes. We know today that those bird viruses can infect the pigs. We also know that if a human virus and a bird virus gets into a pig cell, the different genes can get all shuffled around and exchanged DNA that can result in a new, and maybe even a lethal, virus.

It can't be said with 100% certainty that this is what happened in 1918, but there sure was a flu outbreak that showed up in January of that year that was so bad that the Haskell County's doctor called it into the Public Health Service and the flu was not even a reportable disease. But, this country doctor knew something was not right in his county. He told them almost everyone in the county had lagrippe (flu) or pneumonia.

What made it worse was that several Haskell County men that had already been exposed to the flu went on to Camp Funston. It started out March 4th, one soldier had the flu and was sick. In two weeks 1,100 soldiers were admitted to the army hospital and thousands sick in their barracks because there was no more room in the hospital. Thirty-eight of them died. Infected soldiers probably carried the flu on to other Army camps in the U.S. All in all, 24 of 36 army camps experienced outbreaks. Tens of thousands of soldiers were sickened from the flu before leaving and carrying it overseas to spread there. Back at home, the disease was spreading into the U.S. civilian homes.

You must bear in mind the flu virus is capable of mutating rapidly. It can change enough that the human immune system has trouble figuring out if it has seen it before and deciding if it can attack it from one season to the next.

Our seasonal flu usually will bind just to our upper respiratory tract which is bad enough. That is our nose and throat which makes us miserable, and that is why we can spread it so easily.

In 1918, the virus was a death trap as it infected cells in the upper respiratory tract, spreading it quickly, but the virus also went deep into the lungs, damaging tissue as it went causing viral and bacterial pneumonia. It was a no-win situation.

You will find some researchers that want to say this flu started in Vietnam or China. I have no idea why they want to say that is where it began as I have found no justification to back up their reasoning.

The spring pandemic flu that folks contracted did not alarm anyone as not many were dying, and some just called it the "three-day fever." If they got it, they needed to call themselves Lucky or Blessed. They had no way of knowing at the time but getting a light case of the flu that Spring saved their lives.

People just did not pay attention to the serious warning signs. The people who did die were the so-called healthy young adults.

When July 1918 rolled around, they announced the flu was over. The flu had disappeared entirely, and everyone was happy.

Starting September 1, 1918, things started changing for the worse. The Army Hospital at Camp Devens could hold 1,200 patients. On this day it had 84 patients.

September 7, 1918, a soldier was brought to the hospital screaming when touched and the doctors there diagnosed him with meningitis. September 8, 2018, there were 12 more men brought in with the same symptoms. The doctors changed the diagnosis to the flu.

The flu diagnosis had turned into an explosion! In one day at Camp Devens, there were 1,543 soldiers with the flu. The hospital could hold no more. The doctors and nurses were sick, no cafeteria workers to feed the patients nor the staff, they could not accept any more patients. That left thousands ill and dying in the barracks.

One of the doctors from Deven wrote to one of his colleagues that he had never seen anything like this; the Pneumonia was the worst he had ever seen. They come in and after they have been here only two hours they have dark red spots above their cheeks, then a few hours later there is Cyanosis that starts at the ears and spreads over their entire face. After that, it is only a few hours, and they are dead. There are about one hundred dying each day, and the bodies are piling up as there are no coffins.

Before anyone could blink twice, the flu was everywhere, even in Alaska and in Africa! How did it get to the frozen tundra of Alaska? This flu strain was killing everyone it seemed. You didn't know when you caught it, if you would live or not.

The whole time, the Government was still claiming there was not a problem. The Sedition Act was still in force, and no one could say anything to the contrary about the flu.

September 28th a big 'Liberty Loan' parade had been planned in Philadelphia. Doctors were all saying it needed to be cancelled.
We must remember a crucial fact before we go any further.

The incubation period for the flu is two to three days. That means after you have been around someone contagious you can start to come down with the flu. It holds true for influenza today.
Do NOT forget this fact.

Two days after the big parade, Philadelphia blew up with the flu.

All the while the newspapers were touting "Scientific Nursing Had Stopped the Flu." The truth of the matter was that the nurses had no impact because there were no nurses available. They were all sick or taking care of their own families.

In one day, Philadelphia was seeing 759 people die a day. In six weeks more than 12,000 people died in the city.

In San Antonio, Texas over half the population was sick with the flu. No one could deny it to them. Those sick with the flu were dying within hours of first showing symptoms. It was not just aches and pains or cyanosis. It was foamy blood they were coughing up from their lungs, and they were bleeding from other orifices like their eyes, ears, and nose. The people were not stupid, and the government was not being fair to them. Why else would everyone be out of coffins?

Citizens of the US started not believing anything they were being told.

By the government burying the truth from them, the countries morale collapsed. Society as we know it had begun to fall.

In Philadelphia, people were not taking a step out of their homes. They were so frightened that they may catch the flu. Fear had emptied all the streets. The life of the city had almost come to a dead stop.

There was a third wave that hit in January 1919 that ended in the spring. And then as quick as it came, it was gone, and life started again. Schools started back up; businesses opened, people celebrated that the war is over, and once again there was traffic in the streets.

Experts are still shaking their heads, and all the questions are still not answered about 1918. Some researchers believe that the first wave in the spring of 1918 was just a regular seasonal flu virus that was different from the pandemic strain; but there again, there is evidence abounding that the pandemic virus did have a virulent and a mild strain.

The death toll was historic, and most people who caught the flu did survive. But overall death rate was 2 percent. The age of those who died was abnormal. It is usually the seniors who pass away from the flu. In 1918, it was young adults between ages of 25 to 45. 3.26% were industrial workers, 6% of coal miners, and 23% to 71% of pregnant women died.

Now, if you are a curious person as I am, you are probably wondering why in the world the young, healthy adults died even if they had no antibodies because their immune system should have been able to mount a decent response to the virus, right?

Because young adults do have the hardiest immune systems, and their immune systems were attacking the virus every way humanly possible; there were things like cytokines and toxins that will fight microbes in their healthy bodies, but, unfortunately, the battlefield was inside their lungs.

The "cytokine storms" alone wreaked havoc and further damaged that healthy patient's lung tissue until it looked much like they had been breathing in poison gas. If you have never seen this image, I urge you to look this up. It is unbelievable. There was no way they could take in oxygen and for a virus to reap that much havoc on an organ in such a short time is hard to conceive.

I am going to give you a little extra information here in case you do not have a medical background, so this will make more sense.

A **cytokine** is part of a group of peptides and proteins that can carry needed signals between human cells to control immune responses to infection.

If you start making too many cytokines, like in the instance of when a flu bug comes along and is not familiar with the cytokine, it might cause too many cytokines to be in one place trying to get rid of the flu bug. If that happens it can create a life-threatening situation of inflammation in the surrounding tissue; this is a **cytokine storm**. If the infection it is attacking is in the lungs, the swelling from the cytokines can cause damage that may be permanent. If it lasts a long time, it can stop breathing altogether.

The flu, as whole, can spread easiliy. It is so easy that it is frightening. If you are within 5-6 feet from anyone who is contagious, any time they laugh, talk, sing, or cough, they can spray droplets that are so microscopic so you cannot see them. If they happen to come your direction, they can land on your mucous membranes of your lips, mouth, nasal passages, or eyes and you are then contaminated. Just like that! You are now inoculated as if you had drank the virus yourself.

Chapter Four: 1976 Swine Flu Pandemic Scare

I can remember well the story of my Mother's Director coming into the medical laboratory where she was working in the hematology division that day in 1976 and announcing that everyone was required to take the Swine Flu Vaccine as employees of the hospital. If they did not accept the vaccine, then if they became sick with the flu, they would not be able to collect pay for sick days.

Money was tight for us with her getting out of school that year and just starting her first job. She stood in line with others dreading the thought but got her vaccine along with everyone else. It was the first 'flu' vaccine she had ever taken in my life.

She was so ill that night; She was sure she would not be alive by morning. Now, she was not a whiner, and anyone in my family would tell you the same. Her fever shot up to 103, and she hurt so bad over her entire body that she knew there had never been anything like this in her life! She had chills and was sweating, and yes, she went to work like that the next day and the next and every day she felt a little bit better. It took her a total of five days to finally feel back to her old self again.

Not till forty years later did I learn the mystery that surrounded that 1976 Swine Flu Vaccine that she stood in line to take. In the following paragraphs, I will try to explain what led up to that day and why she and others felt so sick and see if you agree with me.

In February of 1976, there was a recruit at Fort Dix in New Jersey who had fallen ill with what seemed like a flu type illness. The New Jersey State Health Department had identified the part of the isolates which were (H3N2), but there seemed to be a couple of the strains they could not type out in their lab, so they sent them on to Atlanta to the CDC.

When they reached the CDC, they identified them as (H1N1); that was the same virus that had caused the Great Flu Pandemic of 1918! What had they been handed?

Immediately there was a meeting of everyone who was anybody.

The National Institute of Health, the New Jersey Health Department, The Food and Drug Administration, and various members of the military and they even met on a Saturday, and it happened to be on Valentine's Day.

They decided to increase surveillance in Fort Dix and to check all the recruits who became ill to see if any of them had been around pigs. They also determined that blood testing of all recruits there in Fort Dix should be done to determine if the Swine Flu was spreading.

Back at Fort Dix, the blood tests proved that transmission had undoubtedly occurred in more than 200 of their recruits.

The young recruit at Fort Dix died, and four others came down with the flu, and those four did recover by the way.

Almost a month later, on March 10, more groups met to review what they had found at Fort Dix. They felt a Pandemic was indeed possible. At this specific point in time, they knew at least five points of concern:

- Anyone younger than 50 would not have antibodies to this strain of flu
- Since it was spring, it would give enough time to produce a vaccine before the fall season when flu would be at its worst
- At the moment there was another strain floating around (A/Victoria)
- In the past, if they incorporated the current strain of circulating flu with the

new vaccine strain it was usually safe, and the efficacy was typically good
- For years they had included in all the military vaccines the (H1N1) vaccine, and they had never had any adverse effects from it

Some at the meeting thought they should get the vaccine made up immediately and start vaccinating while others thought they should have it made and stockpile the vaccine.

Pay careful attention to the next couple of sentences as I think they are the most important of all in the CDC report.

The pharma companies who made the vaccines had just finished making up all the vaccines for the 1976-1977 flu season. They were DONE. During that time, the flu vaccine was developed by using fertilized hen's eggs that came from a certain kind of hen. Roosters they used for the fertilization process were still available if they were not slaughtered which was what always had been done with them when they were finished with that season's flu vaccines. If this was the case, they COULD NOT start production again for several months.

More top official meetings ensued. Then, out of the blue, there was a proposal that 'recommended,' that the Federal Government should contract with 'private' companies for the United States to procure enough vaccine for our entire population against the Swine Flu. They wanted the Feds to give grants to all the state health departments for their part in organizing and conducting the immunizations as they had planned. Finally, they wanted the H1N1 included in the A/Victoria vaccine that was being given anyway.

A memo followed all the above requests to the White House reminding them of the 1918 Pandemic and that what we were facing carried that potential. President at the time, Gerald Ford called together several respected doctors and scientists that included Jonas Salk and Albert Sabin, so they could hear the proposal. After the meeting, Ford held a press conference and asked Sabin and Salk to speak as well. They announced that this would be happening.

The Swine Flu Vaccine Program had begun.

The cost of this plan was $137 million. In ten weeks, they had vaccinated 45 million people.

The BIG obstacle that lay before them was - not enough vaccine. There were test batches, but they were conducting the most significant field trials they had ever performed with this flu vaccine. The vaccine seemed to be safe, but they soon realized the children were not seroconverting when they received only one dose of the flu vaccine.

Still, yet, they felt good about the fall vaccine season."

Then Ugly #1 started to raise its head.

Instead of getting in bottles of the vaccine, the private contractors said they were not going to take responsibility for any claims for adverse reactions associated with the vaccine. It became a huge worry. What was wrong with the vaccine? The perception of the public whether it be the right vaccine or not, was there and made sure that no matter what occurred when the public was vaccinated or anytime close to it, they would blame the flu vaccine.

Then Ugly #2 showed up in August at an American Legion convention held in Philadelphia. After the CDC's full investigation, it was found to be Legionnaires disease from the water. It didn't matter to the public. They saw it as a way that the government was trying to persuade them to be vaccinated.

Ugly #3 came roaring in like a lion when three senior people died after they had got their flu shot at the same clinic. The investigations could find no commonalities, even Walter Cronkite, as pessimistic as he was, could see the pattern; The entire scenario was just not looking good. All three at the same clinic?

In some of my research, I found 500 people who developed Guillian Barre' Syndrome and in some articles, it goes as high as 3,000 that developed the Syndrome. If you have never known anyone with Guillian Barre', then count yourself as lucky. It is so sad the way the myelin sheaths are stripped of their coating so that the impulses from the brain cannot send the appropriate signals so that someone cannot walk, use their arms and in many cases, cannot breathe without a respirator. It takes months of rehab care for them to regain their strength after many IV's of gamma globulin is given to recoat the myelin sheaths. The process does not happen overnight either. It takes about two weeks or longer for the feeling to start to come back if it does. There were 32 cases of Guillain Barre' that caused death after the vaccine in 1976.

The government paid dearly to the patient's and their families for those affected. No matter what you try to find, there is a lot of talk about this topic, and it is written as so many cases of GBS per 100,000, but CDC never tells you how many hundreds of thousands they are talking about, so you can't figure an exact number. Thank goodness for what news reporters brought out at that time, or we would not know some of what we do.

Center for Disease Control will tell you that when citizens lives are at stake, it is better to make your error on the side of caution. It takes courage to make the choices that must be made at the time. Every decision that affects lives like this will entail benefits and risks.

It is my opinion and my opinion alone, but I feel that in 1976 when they decided to make the vaccine so rapidly that the chickens and roosters were already slaughtered. I think the contract companies were chosen because the hens and roosters were already dead and they were working with live vaccine and that the public was given a live vaccine, not an attenuated (dead) version of the Swine Flu Vaccine.

I believe they were told to use the live virus. I think the private contract companies were told to do this for the common good as there was not the time to use the eggs and make it through the normal process. For this reason, I feel confident that is why the private contract companies did not want to take on the liability of the flu vaccines that were to being given because they knew what they would be providing the public.

Because Gerald Ford and his wife got their flu shots on national TV proves not one thing to me. That could have been saline or a vaccine for the A/Victoria flu strain. We have no way of ever knowing.

Because of the 1976 Swine Flu vaccine, there were several lives interrupted (from what we know at least 532) and some destroyed (the 32 who died). What choices would you have made had you been faced with the same set of circumstances? Would you have taken the Swine Flu Vaccine in 1976? If my Mother had to do it over again, she would not.

Chapter Five: Why World Health Authorities Are Now Worried About The Next Flu Pandemic

When the World Health Authorities become worried, then I become a little more concerned, but I always keep both ears to the floor and start doing my own research.

I am going to begin this story with where this flu seems to be starting and tell you about a hard-working family. The husband is what else, but a corn farmer living in China. The husband is 50 years old, and he has one son, and his wife came down with vomiting and some fatigue in March of 2017. Since she was just under the weather, they went to the local herbalist who they could afford because of Yin; the husband only makes $550 a month.

Unfortunately, the herbs did not work, and they had to hire someone to drive them twenty miles to a hospital. At first, they diagnosed her with ulcers and gave her medicine for colic and something the Chinese use for fevers. Two days passed and she was no better, and they placed her in the ICU. One day later the doctors told the husband his wife had H7N9. Yin's wife was the one who stayed at home taking care of her elderly mother and worked out in the cornfields when they needed her. But, a few days before she had walked almost an hour to the open air live poultry market and came home with five chickens that were still alive.

They figured out too late what was wrong with Yin's wife and she died. Yin's hospital bills were astronomical, and he is suing the hospital for not diagnosing his wife in time to save her life. The hospital has counter sued him for his debts that he owes them. Debts he will never be able to pay if he continues to make $550 a month.

2013 was the first time H7N9 had spread from birds to humans. Since that time, we have had five, yes, I said FIVE waves of this deadly virus. The last wave was in October 2016. When September 2017 rolled around, there had been 764 humans infected. Recently the number has risen to 1,589, and 616 of them have died. That, my friend, is a 40% mortality rate. I am sure you agree with me that YOU do not wish to be a statistic.

As of this writing, the only way to contract this deadly virus is by exposure to an infected animal. However, if H7N9 decides to mutate (which is nothing to this virus) and develop the ability to pass from human to human, it can kill millions.

The idea of a pandemic like that of 1918 has medical researchers worried.

What is so terrible is that the live bird markets located in China have been told to shut down for years, but they have not listened to the repeated warnings of what is happening. It is how they make their livings. The government does not seem to make much effort in enforcing the laws either.

You might see as you walk through these markets people with dozens of cages stacked up that are full of all kinds of poultry and fowl and most of the time it is outside what they call their home or hut. If you pick out the chicken you want; the chicken guy with his market will, right there in front of you, slit their throats and toss their bodies in a filthy tall ceramic pot and then wait for the flailing of the birds to calm down. When the birds have calmed, he will dunk them in boiling water (that was already used over and over). He will then toss them into a type of feather picker and tell you no picture taking because he knows it is all against the law.

I realize that China has their hands full, but a couple of years ago, there was on the morning news 16,000 pigs floating in the Yangtze River. It is my understanding that the people were told by their government it was safe to drink from that river as the pigs had died of the flu. The next day over 12,000 ducks were found dead and floating in the same river with the pigs. What gives here? What happened and why were they thrown into the river? Who was responsible? What caused the ducks to die?

It has been 3-4 years now that China bought out Smithfield Pork here in the United States. The pork does not have to pass FDA inspection when they bring in their Pork products to the United States. For that reason, I do not buy Smithfield products anymore. I cannot believe our government gave blessings to this sale. China injects their swine with what the U.S. considers toxins that we do not use in the U.S. We have no idea if the pig that was butchered (and brought to your grocery store) was dead from slaughter or illness. I may be alone in my boycott, but I will not let my family be a part of the contamination that can come into the United States by this method.

Health authorities in China feel that shutting down the live-bird markets would help contain a flu outbreak of the avian strain. You may remember in 1997 when the H5N1 virus was spreading from mainland China into Hong Kong. Authorities there took draconian measures and shut down all the cities live poultry markets and killed 1.6 million chickens to prevent a major flu epidemic.

During the winter of 2016-2017 colleagues were heard saying they were 'startled' to find that the H7N9 virus that had not been a pathogen to the birds before and now it had started killing them! It was a virus mutation that was something new, and the lab found out about it before the vendors were saying a word.

Think about it though, in 2015, H5N2, a flu strain broke out in the United States and spread throughout the entire country and resulted in the slaughtering of 48 million birds.

What makes China different from other countries, is it that the people, the poultry, and the other livestock all live close together in one small hut. The chickens and pigs can run in and out of their living quarters. The swine can have both human flu and bird flu at the same time, and this makes them a "petri dish" or a "mixing vessel" that will let the viruses come together and exchange their DNA and go crazy mutating and creating a new but more deadly form of flu than ever.

If I had not been in healthcare for the time I have and certified as an Infection Control Practitioner, I would be going through life not worrying about what was out there. I would not be opening any public doorknob with a paper towel. I would not keep germex throughout my home. I would not continue to hold several gallons of chlorox in my garage and multiple bottles of small chlorine tablets in my laundry room cabinets.

But when you know the threats that exist, it does make you seem a little paranoid and yes to some sound a bit crazy I suppose. Public Health Experts and Scientists both agree that it is not 'if' a flu pandemic breaks out, it is 'when.' They are calling it the 'Plague.'

When the 'Plague' happens, and we are buried in the throes of the first days of this terrible pandemic that has been thrust upon us, there will be many decisions that have to be made by our government and scientists. Some not so popular with the public.

They will be about treatment, containment, and prophylaxis and the people once again will get limited information. They still will fear that if they communicate to the public the real message that it will provoke panic and fear. But if they do not report enough, people will not take it seriously, and the number who die will be much higher. No matter what, they will not trust the government and what they are saying. But worse than not trusting our government, they will not believe what the media has to report.

Chapter Six:
Where, When, And How Will The Next Major Flu Epidemic Hit Us?

We all want to know that burning question. I for one want to know which direction to look and what age group is it most likely to kill this time.

The Flu Experts would probably tell us that H5N1 which is the "bird flu." will be the ONE. So far it has not been able to be transferred from human to human, but you have had to get it from the animal.

Don't be relaxing so fast; any flu can change in the blink of an eye, and all of sudden it can be spread via sneezing, coughing, talking, laughing, or singing and attaching itself to your tracheal, eyes, or nasal membranes just like the seasonal flu does every year.

Here is an excellent example for you:

Last year, after my flu vaccine like ALWAYS, I was at work. It had been well past the two weeks for antibodies to develop. There was a potential new hire for interviewing that morning. The young girl was sitting across the desk from me coughing and hacking, obviously very ill. She was asked by me, "So how long have you been sick?" She replied, "I have the flu. I have been in bed all weekend, and I have 103 degrees of temperature right now." All the time she is coughing and blowing her nose repeatedly. Immediately this Manager donned a mask, put on gloves and told her we needed to reschedule her appointment. She was told to give me a call when she got well. She was worried she would not get the job. She was assured that her tenacity was admired, but in the light of the flu season, she needed to get well first. Her job appointment interview was safe. Out came the disinfectant wipes and everything that could be wiped down was cleaned. The entire office was fumigated with disinfecting spray. There was gargling with salt water. Scrubbing of self-till raw was also carried out. At that time no one had been notified that the flu vaccine was only 42% effective.

Worry about the exposure did not last long. Two days later it was like a truck had run over my chest, 103 degrees of fever and taking Tylenol and Ibuprofen every four hours alternating them could only get my temp down to 102. I genuinely did not care if I lived. It hurt to raise my head and to move any part of my body. I had to admit; it was official, this was the flu. I was officially a casualty from the new hire in the interview. There were 2 ½ large boxes of Kleenexes used in that one week. No one was allowed in our home. Quarantining myself in my house was the best for everyone.

Each of those days was 72 hours long, and the crazy dreams with the fevers were just that, crazy. After three days, my temperature each day started going down some. They were staying around 102. That was better than 103.

My one question was where had it attached to me? It had to be my mouth or my nasal area when the new hire talked and sprayed droplets that I breathed in or when I talked, and she coughed or spoke at the same time.

The researchers tell us that even mutated N5H1, after just five mutations, could latch itself to the cells of our tracheal and nasal passages, and this for all of us, is grim news.

They tell us that Surveillance is ramping up for the virus throughout all of Asia in the Southeastern section. Bangladesh is supposedly on the front line.

The ones who are researching are not sitting on their thumbs waiting for the Big One to hit, they keep working on a new prototype if you will, a so-called starter vaccine, so they can test it against any new flu strain.

Since it takes at the minimum of four to six months to develop a vaccine, we must remember that some countries will not have the scientific resources, the medical prowess, nor the infrastructural resources at hand no matter what to take care of their people.

I guess I am an impatient person. They have put many men on the moon, people working on a space station, and they are about to send people to Mars, but can't come up with a vaccine in a shorter time frame than four to six months. Something is just not right. That time frame would let the flu pandemic be over with, and everyone going back to their lives.

The way in which vaccine is made seems to be outdated, and they haven't seemed to have changed it much in the past 70 years. They are still using the hens' eggs approach in which to replicate the virus.

We do find out from the Coalition for Epidemic Preparedness Innovations however that there have been some recent scientific advances that were much needed. These advancements are racing ahead with vaccines supposedly developing at a much faster rate.

They are using a Genomic technique to map out the RNA and DNA of a newly discovered pathogen, then genetically engineer that same RNA or DNA, and Mass produce it and have it ready to inject to humans. Once injected into the human body then it would lead to the production of antibodies prepared to fight the flu. We would come to know this as a DNA vaccine. It would shorten the vaccine process by 24 weeks. AMAZING!

Sounds great, does it not? But then there is bureaucracy and red tape, and that will take another ten years because of Food and Drug Administration Guidelines.

Right now, feelings are that the next flu pandemic will most likely come from the open-air bird markets in China.

Someone, anyone, could contract the flu, maybe a visitor or a traveler that then catches a plane to New York. This person has exposed everyone in the airport and on the plane. Once landing in New York, they expose many in the airport. They then hail a cab, all the while the traveler is feeling worse and can barely hold up his head. They expose the cab driver to the flu that they now have the full-blown version, so they are very contagious. They arrive at their hotel where he is greeted by the doorman and the hotel guest services; two more are exposed. He makes it to his room where he falls across his bed because he cannot take one more step. That is where they find his dead body two days later. All the people he has encountered on his way, he has exposed to the flu virus he was carrying, and they unknowingly started feeling bad a day or two later at which time they were able to start spreading the flu virus themselves not realizing they had the flu.

This is exactly how a flu pandemic could begin. Sounds like a movie plot but this one is even scarier.

In the U.S. Alone, if a flu pandemic were to start, there would be several events that would happen almost immediately.

1) Everyone would be demanding medical attention and going to their doctor's office or the Emergency Room and spreading more flu virus around.

2) You would see a decrease in demand for restaurant services, hotel rooms, and probably mass transit

3) You will see few people at public events, there will be very few people out shopping.

4) Employees would not be showing up to work because they are ill, or they are caring for family causing lost revenue for their families;

it would generate impaired daily business functions, lower business revenues, and lower household incomes. It could just as well influence revenue from tourism and restrictions on trade.

If you were not sick and you went on to work, on your way there, you might notice that you are meeting very few cars on your drive. You pull into the gas station, but they are sold out, and no one is at the gas station. It is locked, and a sign is on the door that says, "Closed till further notice." You decide to go to the grocery store to pick up a few things to have at work in the break room for your lunches this week. At the grocery store, you notice there are very few workers, the shelves are almost bare, there is no fresh produce to choose from, and when you check out with a can of tuna, the checker has on a mask.

You drive on to work, and the building is almost empty. You see a co-worker from another floor. You ask the co-worker from upstairs how things are going and they tell you they are not feeling too good and they are going home. You notice that your computer will not work, and you call the IT department. There is no answer, but the answering machine says that the IT department is closed until further notice. Everyone is out sick. There is no one on your floor but you. Your computer does not work. You might as well go back home. But, you need the income. What choice do you have? How are you not sick? You head back home.

When you arrive back to your home, you should turn on your tv and listen to the news. They should be giving directions as to what everyone should be doing.

Everyone should have at least two weeks of supplies on hand at home in the event of a flu pandemic. Be aware however that the epidemic may last for several months. In your stockpile, make sure you have bottled water, plenty of your medications, food, and facemasks.

Make sure you wash your hands often and use soap and water. If you have no water, use an alcohol-based hand gel. If you cough or sneeze, be sure to cover your mouth and nose and get rid of your Kleenex immediately.

Keep a good supply of masks at home. You do not have to buy the expensive kind of N95 masks. The typical surgical masks will work fine for the flu. You are protecting yourself from droplets. Keep a mask with you at all times and in your home keep a box of them on hand.

Wearing one this year when in public after finding out the flu vaccine of 2018 was only 10% effective is also a smart move. I do not trust others when they are sick to stay home. Most people are not responsible for illness and do not take the precautions that are necessary.

You will see that since the flu strains all affect the respiratory system, if there should be a pandemic, that many will need ventilators and there will not be enough for everyone. The hospitals will run out of rooms to keep patients in the hospital.

Worse than that, there will not be enough staff and physicians to care for those that are in the hospital because they or their family will be ill as well.

There are some things that we do know however that our government has worked hard and long to prepare. It was done with the Congressional Research Service and the Department of Defense planning for a Flu Pandemic.

We already know that we cannot predict when a pandemic will occur as they are unpredictable. We can take a look at the history of the past epidemics and see what happened then, but it in no way can be used to assume that will be what will happen this time during a pandemic.

According to the Federal Government here is a list of their planning efforts:
- We know that everyone will be

susceptible to the virus.

- If it can be transmitted between people, then we have an imminent pandemic.

- We can expect the attack rate to be at least 30 % of the entire population during the total time of the pandemic. We will see the highest number of ill in kids that are school aged, and it will decline with age. As for working adults, we are looking at an average of 20 % that will come down with the flu. (This is very hard for me to believe as it was MUCH higher than that in 1918 and number one says that EVERYONE will be susceptible to the virus. Tamiflu is becoming resistant, and if that proves right with the next pandemic, we have nothing to defend ourselves.)

- There will be some that are infected but never develop enough symptoms to bother them. Even though patients do not show signs or they show a few symptoms they can still transmit the flu to someone else.

- We do not know how many people will seek care from their doctor. In previous epidemics, about 50% of people who became ill would seek attention. Since there are antiviral medications available now, there may be more people in to see their physicians.

- Those seeking care will probably depend on the severity of the patient's illness. The groups anticipated in the next pandemic for severity of disease are more than likely to be inclusive of immuno-suppressive medical conditions, chronic health problems, pregnant women, the elderly, and infants.

- We also know that the absenteeism in the workplace and schools will depend on how severe the pandemic will become over time. It could reach as high as 40%. That being said, if schools are closed, and households are quarantined this will probably help to decrease rates.

- We know that the time between exposure to the flu and you start having symptoms is about two days.

- People who become infected can shed the flu virus and transmit the infection to others for a half day to one day before you even have symptoms. The most significant time of viral shedding that you can transfer to others is during the first two days you are sick. Children are the best at spreading the illness as they do not contain their secretions as well.

- People who are infected can transmit the flu to about two more people. It is only an average. (I do not agree with this number. It mainly depends on how many people you come in contact with at the time.) I feel confident the young lady I was interviewing spread the flu to at least 25-50 people because she talked to so many on her way to my office.

- Epidemics usually last 6-8 weeks in communities.

- Pandemics will last months around the world.

- There will be multiple waves when the illness becomes active again, and each time it may last 2-3 months. The worst and most significant waves are usually in the fall and winter, and this is generally due to everyone staying inside because it is cold outside.

We must also consider other areas as we plan and prepare for what may happen in the event of a flu pandemic:

- There will probably be some disruptions and restrictions that will slow down supplies that are essential to everyday living. It can mean groceries, paper products, medicines, fuel, office supplies, etc.

- School closures and what you will do with your children while the schools are closed.

- Businesses that directly serve the public face to face will see an abrupt drop in customers and income to their business, while online stores and telephone orders will see sharp increases.

- You will find that Banks and other financial groups reducing direct contact with their customers. They will urge you to make electronic transfers, use the ATMs, and drive up tellers instead of coming into the bank itself.

- Municipal infrastructure will cause you to find some delays in your service to your routine utilities.

If there were a Pandemic today; could the Life Insurance Industry Survive the Avian Flu?

They seem to think that they can. How?

They say that if there were a severe pandemic like that of 1918 that it could cost the Life Insurance companies up to $155 billion. However, they feel that amount would be made up within the next year by people who would sign up for life insurance after experiencing the Flu Pandemic. Do you agree with that statement? I am wondering who would have the money to buy life insurance if the pandemic left our country in a recession as it well could.

Chapter Seven: The Department Of Defense During A Flu Pandemic

There are countries that even with the entire world engulfed in a pandemic would take the advantage to do even more damage than what is already being done by the flu. Expect anything.

Our government is ahead of the game on all points I can assure you. If it should happen, we must be patient.

A couple of examples are: if they should shut down our entire power grid for the country; another is if they add on a biological warfare agent, and as if that would not be enough if they could launch a massive cyber attack.

The Defense Department will be working closely with the Civil Authorities. We would likely see the National Guard in our neighborhoods. Below is a list of the few responsibilities they will try to be available to assist with:

- Laboratory diagnostics and disease surveillance
- Providing transport of vaccines, supplies, pharmaceuticals, blood products, medical equipment, and diagnostic devices
- Evacuation of injured and ill
- Treating patients
- Tracking and processing patients
- Supplying federal, state, local, and tribal agencies with base and installation support
- Overseeing and controlling the movement in and out of areas, across borders, with the affected populations
- Providing support to law enforcement
- Providing support for quarantine enforcement
- Assist in restoring public utilities that have been damaged
- Provision of morgue services

Usually, the requirement of a morgue is where they bring in refrigerated semi-truck trailers, and they place the bodies in them until it can be decided what they will be able to do with the bodies.

Their support for quarantine enforcement is when citizens will not stay in their homes as they have been asked to do for the containment of the flu. Once your home is quarantined, you must remain inside no matter the circumstance. It does not matter if you think you are going stir crazy, you MUST stay in your home. That is what the National Guard is there to enforce. To stop the spread of infection, you must cooperate. It is for a good reason.

    I know you have seen movies on TV that make the National Guard look like the bad guys and they are there to kill you, or that is how the movies portray them at times. That is not the case in the event of a pandemic. They are there to help. If you have problems with them, it is because you have done something you should not. It is your job to cooperate.

Chapter Eight:
So, How Do We Move Forward?

Most of us who watch the news and are obsessed with such things as infections, pandemics and epidemics know that the drug Tamiflu prescribed when you have the flu has not been effective against the flu strain circulating in 2009.

Scientists tell us that it is not the overuse of Tamiflu, but because of a spontaneous genetic mutation. I must wonder about this fact.

Again, my opinion, drinking water will do about as much good. I have good friends who are pharmacists who will tell you the same thing.

Dr. Matthew Faiman from Cleveland Clinic is quick to respond to Tamiflu. He will tell you that of course, everyone wants to get 'over' the flu quicker. If you would start taking it within 48 hours of when your symptoms start (this is extremely important) and if you are lucky you will maybe get well one day quicker of a seven to ten-day sick spell. Tamiflu's mechanism of stopping the flu virus is to prevent it from reproducing so your body's immune system can kill it.

Another reason most do not take Tamiflu is that it is so expensive, and most insurances no longer pay for it. Tamiflu may cost you just for the copay $75 if you have insurance, and if you have to pay without insurance, it may run you $210 or more and for it to knock off one day of the flu? Is it worth that kind of money? Now, if you have my kind of luck, that day would probably be the day when you are starting to feel better anyway, so why spend it?

For me, I will be using Elderberry Syrup, Bryonia, and Gelsemium with Gelsemium being my first line of defense. I have researched Elderberry, and it too stops bacteria and viruses from replicating. With the success rate of Gelsemium during 1918, I would take it before I would buy Tamiflu and 'hope' that the Tamiflu might work.

So, how close do I think we are to a vaccine specific to this possible flu they predict is coming?

First, they are not sure which one will hit, but they believe it is N1H1. We will see. We will also see if a vaccine can be made in time before the pandemic reaches us.

The perfect result would be to develop a vaccine for all seasons. Yes, you read that the right way. They want to design a universal vaccine for the flu that will work for any flu that comes along and somewhere along the way they mentioned they wanted to make it viable for ten years so that is how often we would have to get the vaccine. I would be all for that if it worked and if it was effective against all the different strains of flu out there.

If someone could take a microscopic flu virus and cut a cross-section of it, it would resemble a little ball that has studs in it that looks like drumsticks (more like a straight sewing pin with a round pearl head on it) and some spikes. The ball itself would be hollow on the inside. The round pearl thing that is on the outside is neuraminidase, known as the part NA or N. The spikes, also on the outside, are the hemagglutinin, that is known as the part HA for H.

Bear with me for a minute as I explain.

You will find there are 18 different subtypes of the hemagglutinin described and there are 11 different subtypes of the neuraminidase that make up flu virus strains. The Flu A strains (ones that usually cause the pandemics) get named by combining the initals of the neuraminidase and the hemagglutinin they have on their surface.

The Pandemic in 1918 was H1N1, in 1957 it was the H2N2, then in 1968, it was H3N2. In all of these, you can have mutations happen all the time, and especially so if the avian virus makes it into swine and other animals.

The hemagglutinin is that portion of the flu virus which causes it stick to cells inside your lungs and turns them into virus factories that make even more viruses. Since the hemagglutinin is on the outside, that is what our immune system will react to but since the virus always mutates, the antibodies made by our immune system this year will probably not be the ones to protect us for flu strains that will show up in the future.

What scientist want to do is to make a vaccine that is a section of this virus that will never change.

That would be from the sticklike stem. They felt it could take care of many virus strains. But, there was a problem with that theory. The flu virus meets with the hemagglutinin head first.

In 2013, they took the head off of an H1 hemagglutinin and then replaced it with a head from a hemagglutinin of a separate branch of a flu virus family tree. It was a strain that affected animals and not humans. Researchers later developed a substitution that worked. The hemagglutinin did provoke an immune response, and it worked on the lab animals by protecting them from the flu. Now a Phase I trial has just started for humans.

We also have the scientist Jeffrey Taubenberger who reconstructed the 1918 flu virus. He is Chief of the Viral Pathogenesis of the National Institute of Allergy and Infectious Diseases. Other flu vaccine researchers consider his methods as unorthodox, but it does seem to be going somewhere. He does not feel that immunity to the stalk is the magic bullet. He believes in Virus-Like Particles (VLP). This method is already being used in Hepatitis B and HPV vaccines.

If this method has already worked for other viruses, why would this approach for the flu virus seem unorthodox to others, except maybe he is ahead of their game? Who knows?

To create their initial version of what they hoped to be a universal vaccine, they used particles of hemagglutinins from four different strains of flu that had been the cause of past pandemics. They then made a cocktail vaccine hoping it would provide better protection than the seasonal vaccines.
It worked in mice against flu strains from those four hemagglutinins they used and against other strains they didn't. Taubenberger doesn't have any idea how it worked with such a broad immunity.

What he would like to do is give a shot early in life, with periodic boosters.

There are other universal vaccines in the works, and whichever one winds up be the 'successful one' and who knows, they may all work. They will all face the same story. No matter what, the vaccine is still a science, and you still have all the burdensome regulations to get it approved, then the manufacturing process and the marketing that goes with it.

When you think about all of that, a universal vaccine will face challenges that are entirely separate from the scientific ones.

The current flu vaccine given brings in more than $3 billion per year worldwide. Why would Big Pharma want to find a one-time universal vaccine and keep them from raking in this amount of money every year? There is no incentive for pharma companies to invest in research and to develop a comprehensive vaccine.

Because, where we stand now if a pandemic like that of 1918 would occur, to halt or try to curb the flu rates would require different strategies for vaccination. Viruses are mutating away, and the process of vaccine development seems to be crawling at a snail's pace and tripped up by all the bureaucracy and red tape that you must endure before it can ever be brought to the light of day and used.

Since there are no vaccines and it looks like it will be years before there will be any, if they do ever show up we need to be prepared as nations.

Our global economy, in about every direction you look with every aspect of commerce, will be affected. A pandemic would be a severe shock to our worldwide network and could have a negative impact on business and trade throughout the entire world. Economists who have analyzed basing a severe pandemic likened to that of 1918 say that it could lead us into a significant economic recession.

Even though there have been plans made in the event, when there is a pandemic that shows up on the horizon, there are still some very fundamental concerns:

- There will always be a lack of available vaccine for use

- There will not be capabilities of the nations to distribute medical equipment and get out vaccines.

- We will run out of gloves, masks, and anti-viral medications.

- No federal monies to pay for the underinsured people coming to emergency rooms that request treatment.

- Not enough extended sick leave for workers so they will stay home when they are sick or could become infected.

- Not enough funding with workers compensation for those workers who became ill while working in their job roles.

- Need to work on strategies for sensible policies to include school closings and to limit public gatherings.

- Preparing on how to inform the public.

- There may be Gaps in 'continued care' after the patient goes home during the time of a pandemic due to lack of resources.

Even hospitals do not keep large quantities of stock and supplies; instead, they use what is called a just-in-time system, and the products are made and shipped when they are needed and requested by the hospital.

Most countries look to their government to have plans readied to deal with disasters and pandemics. But a pandemic, such as that of 1918, would quickly overstretch all monies on the federal, state and local levels, leaving each person on their own to survive.

If it comes to a flu epidemic, it will be a fact that the first one that comes in needing a ventilator, gets the ventilator, and after that, unless another hospital nearby can have an available ventilator, you will probably be drawing your last breath within a few hours.

Hospitals do not have an arsenal of respirators because they are expensive to buy, upkeep and maintain. You can rent them, but when it comes to an epidemic or pandemic, then there would likely not be any available.

The absolute, hardest part is telling the family that their loved one will not be getting a ventilator.

It is hard to understand how people will take chances when they are told that they must wear a mask and should wear goggles, wash their hands frequently and keep away from crowds and especially do not go around people who are sick. These are the very people who do not heed to one word that has been said to them. It is for their protection, and they act like they will not contract the flu or whatever death threatening disease you do not want them to contract.

With my background and experience, I always keep a careful eye on the CDC and WHO websites. My home will continue to keep on hand the natural medications spoken about in an earlier chapter. There will be on hand plenty of gloves and face masks and eye covers and a food supply to last for over two weeks. There will be no problem with not going out to the public.

My vigilance is already heightened because of my trust in this years and last years flu vaccines. I am sorely disappointed in the efficacy of 42% for 2016, 11% for 2017 and 10% for 2018. What road are we heading down? Is it the manufacturer or is it true that the mutation is that quick?

It makes me wonder why I bother to get the flu vaccine every year.

One must wonder if there will ever be a universal flu vaccine and if Big Pharma maybe has something to do with it. Believe me; they probably wouldn't mind interfering with its progress since it affects their bottom line.

They have enough lobbyist on the Hill in Washington D.C. to pay everyone to do as they please.

So, we have learned that if a pandemic should come along, we should be prepared with primary measures and use good common sense:

- Consider quarantining your family

- Have the minimum of two weeks supplies of food and water in your home, include your pets in this as well.

- Inventory and secure all the medications you will need for that time frame.

- Be prepared in case the electricity or heat should go off.

- If you are required for some reason to go out in public, wear a mask and protective gloves.

- Keep plenty of disinfectant on hand at home.

This is the most efficient way you can provide for your families safekeeping. Keep their health and well being in mind at all times and that will get you through the time you have to spend in quarantine.

Final Words

I hope this book has given you more wisdom in the area of the flu, production of vaccines, and flu epidemics and pandemics than before you read it.

If you allow yourself, you will easily be able to find someone in your family that lived during the Great Flu Pandemic of 1918. They may have passed on by now, but if they lived through that time, you would know they were one of the lucky ones.

This book should be dedicated to the men and women who sacrificed so much in 1918 to help others so that they may live and for those who gave of themselves in supporting those in their time of need.

1918 should be a lesson that we all learn from, for history always repeats itself. In this case, I think it will be sooner than later.

Lastly, if you found this book beneficial, then I'd like to ask you for a favor. Would you be so kind to leave a review for this book on Amazon? It would be very much appreciated

D.W. Graeme

www.ingramcontent.com/pod-product-compliance
Lightning Source LLC
Chambersburg PA
CBHW070401230526
45471CB00006B/2660